SO YOU'RE HAVING A BABY
HOW SHOULD YOU
TELL PEOPLE

Written By: Sam Hall

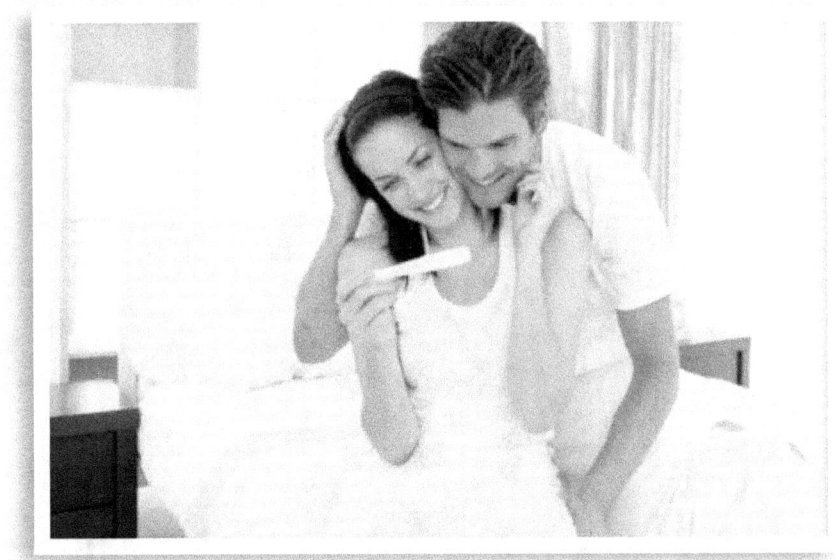

The little blue/pink/green line is there! After months and months of trying to conceive, you and your partner are welcoming a new life into your family. Or, after a few days of wondering where your period went, you've got a bundle on the way. Or, you've been feeling a bit icky and tired lately and just now put the pieces together on why you're so exhausted all of the time.

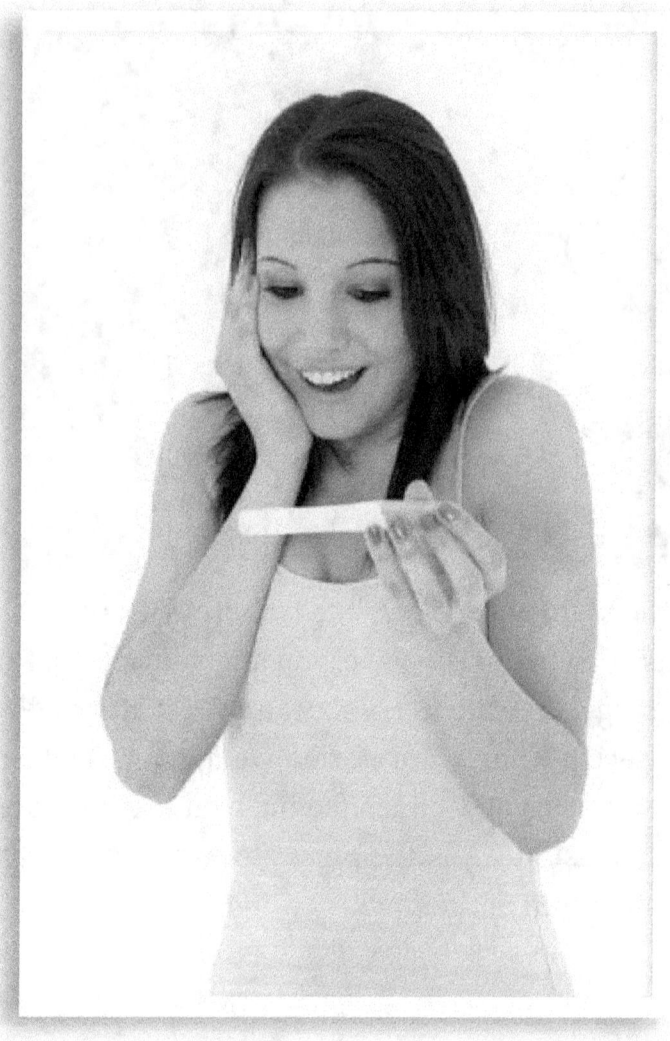

Any way you slice it, you've got some big news, and it's burning a hole in your lips as you try to figure out how to navigate the life changing words. How do you tell everyone?

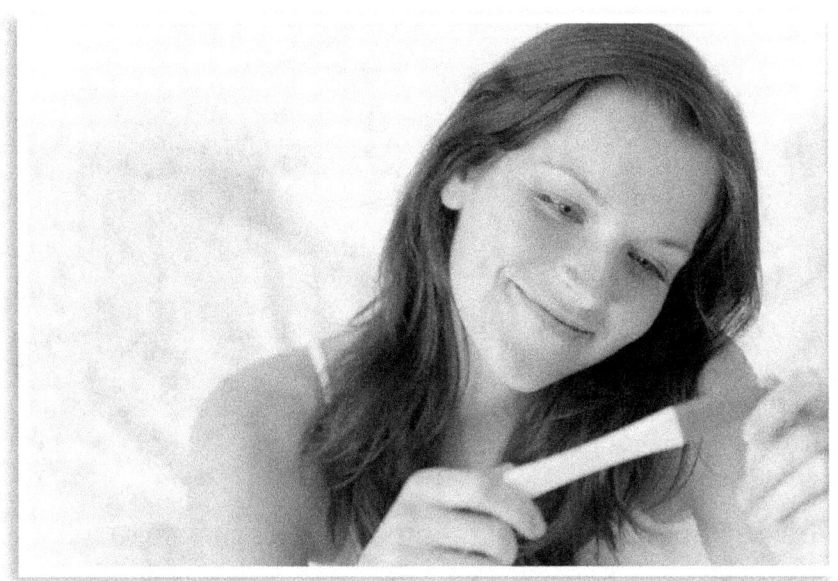

There are several groups of people in your life that need to know this news, and many women elect for a staggered approach when revealing this information. The first step is to get a confirmation of pregnancy from your doctor, who will do an initial scan and determine important things like when the baby is due and if the development is on track.

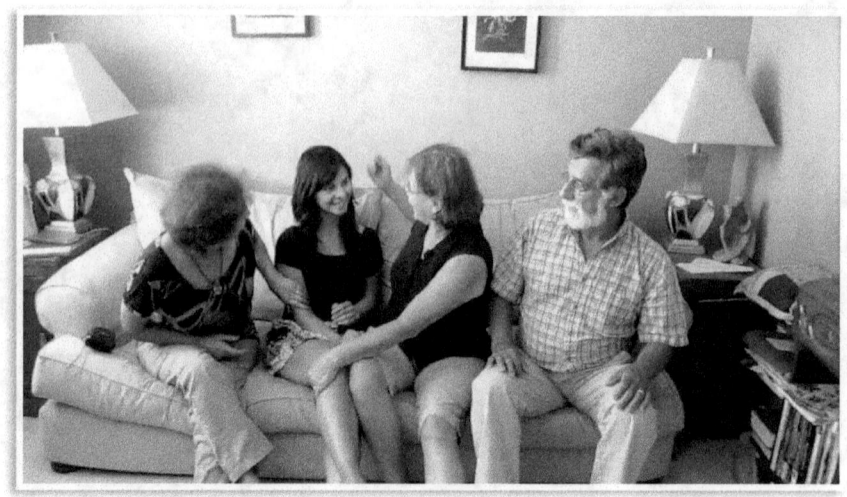

Now the fun begins. Most mothers-to-be choose to tell their families right away, as soon as the pregnancy is confirmed. After all, you have to tell somebody, and your family is the most likely to share your excitement about the new bundle of love. They are, after all, receiving a great gift and a new baby to spoil, without any of the midnight wakings to go with it.

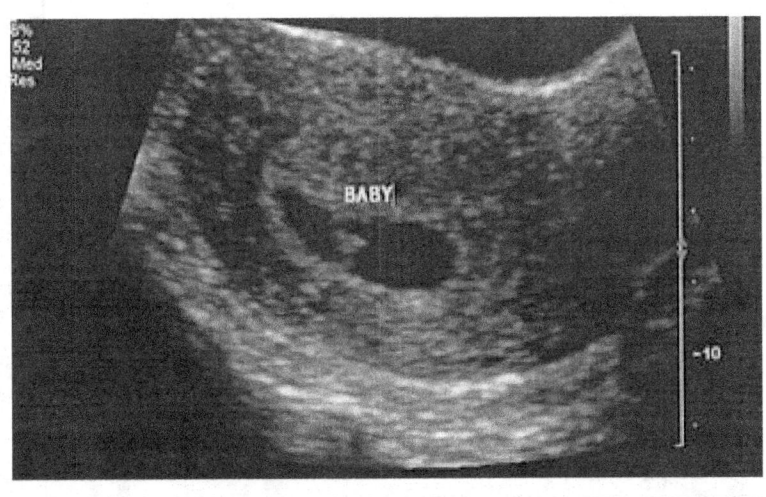

The announcement for your family should be personalized, since you likely aren't ready to share your news with the whole world. If you are far away from them, a card in the mail to grandma and grandpa is a very cute keepsake for them to treasure forever, perhaps with a copy of the baby's first scan. If you're on your second or third, try giving the older sibs to be shirts or signs so that they can announce the pregnancy and be part of the excitement.

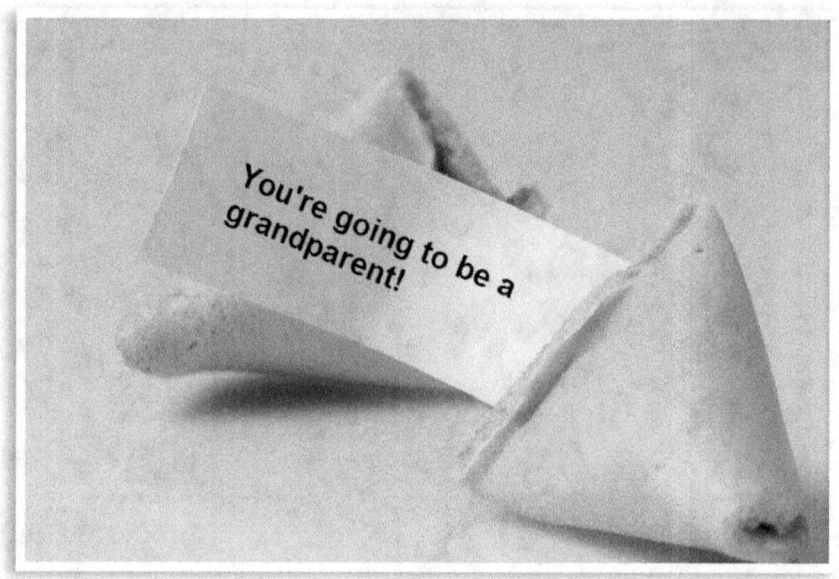

A tech-savvy mum might choose to do a video for her folks. If you think this might be the way to go, check out the internet for some fun ideas. Elaborate song parodies are the latest trend, but having a soon to be older sibling announce it to the family can be just as heartwarming. Make sure that the video is unlisted, so that no prying eyes can find it before you're ready. Also, if you don't want it shared, you need to stipulate that up front before grandma outs you to the whole internet!

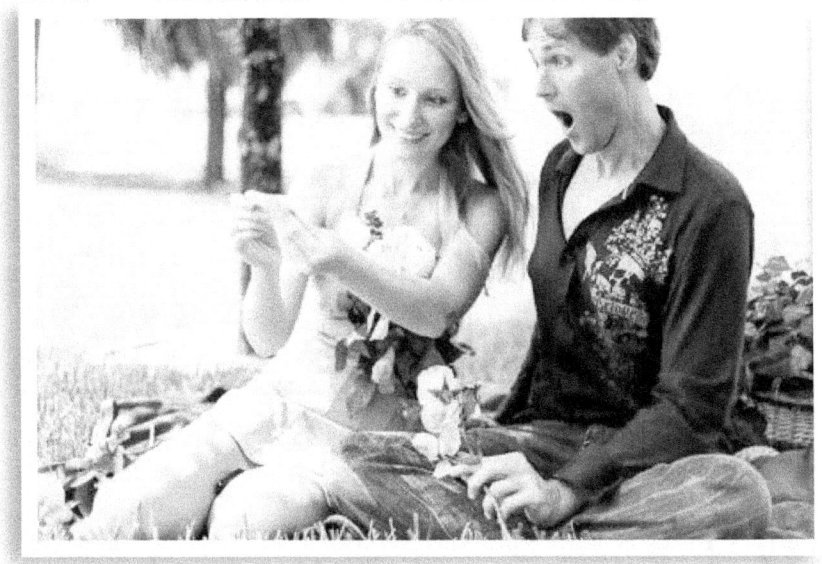

If your family is anything like mine, you'll only have to tell your closest relatives. You can leave distant cousins to find out within the hours that it will take for the 10-20 excited phone calls to reach their ears, especially if you haven't seen them in a while.

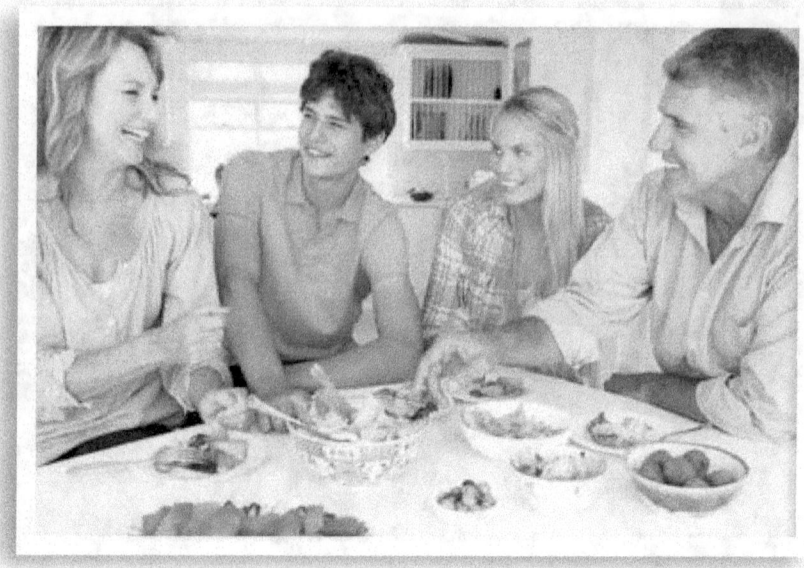

After you inform your relatives, decide who amongst your friends is on a need to know basis. Many women follow the rule that the general public isn't informed about their pregnancy until the second trimester, when the placenta is in place and complications are less common.

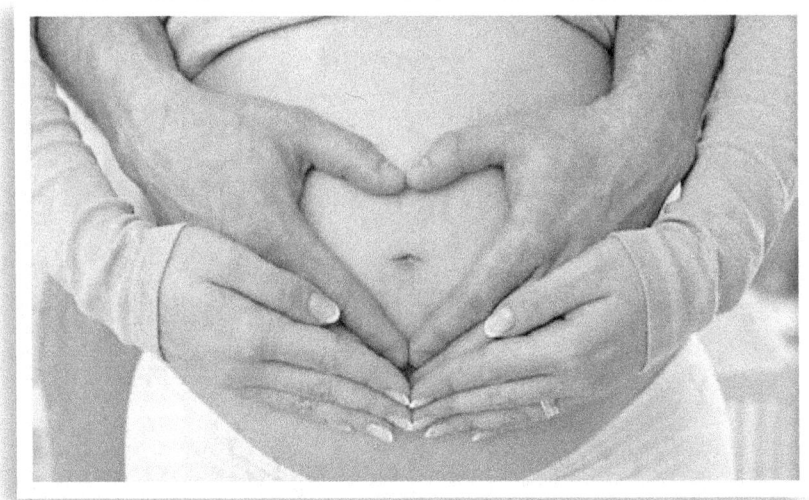

A more recent movement aimed at encouraging women to celebrate pregnancy earlier, and grieve about pregnancy loss more publicly, is currently storming the internet. Make the decision that is right for you, and don't ever feel pressured to tell more people than you are ready for. Even if they find out three or four months in, they've got half a year to get used to the idea before a baby enters the equation.

Of course, there are dozens of cute ways to jazz up your big reveal, and taking the time to be creative will make a big memory for your family! We've listed a ton of great ideas below, which you can film or photograph to share when the big news goes public.

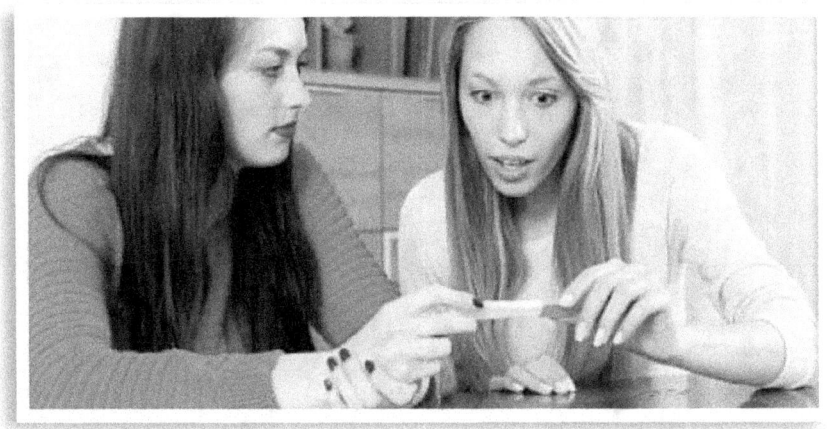

The most fun way to tell your closest friends may be to gather everyone for a brunch and spring it on at once, especially if you have a group of close knit friends that warrant knowledge at the same time. Again, if you're of the mind that this needs to be under wraps from the public, make sure they know this going in. Any way you do it, these announcements are more fun in person so you can fully enjoy the moment!

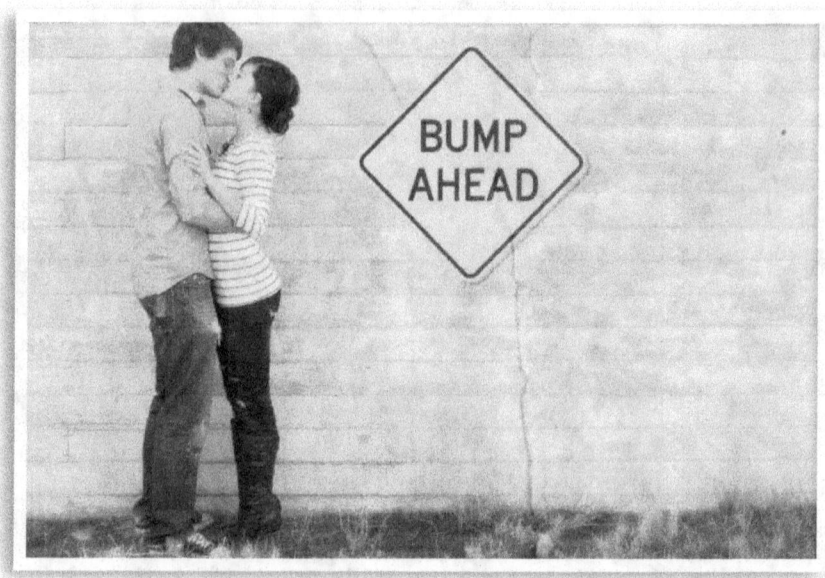

Depending on the nature of your community (i. e. several of your friends know people you work with), work should be the next on the docket. You'll have a lot to figure out when it comes to your job, but don't assume that this means your employer will react negatively. Everybody loves babies, or at the very least understands that this is an exciting development in your life.

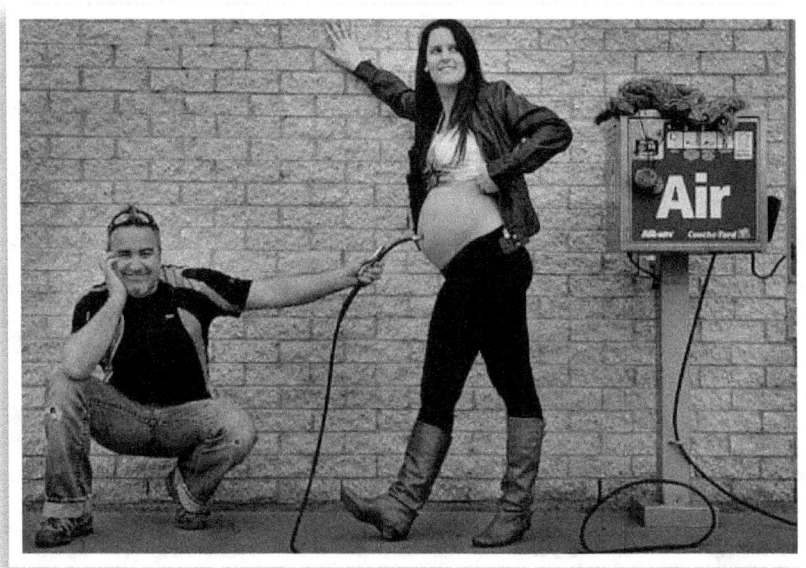

Your work announcement will probably be the least fun of all, but you still need to carefully consider how to handle it. Unfortunately you need to do a little bit of reading up on your company's policies and your rights in the workplace, as this will inevitably come up. Be sure to have a proposed plan in place so that your boss knows you've thought this through, and stick to your guns.

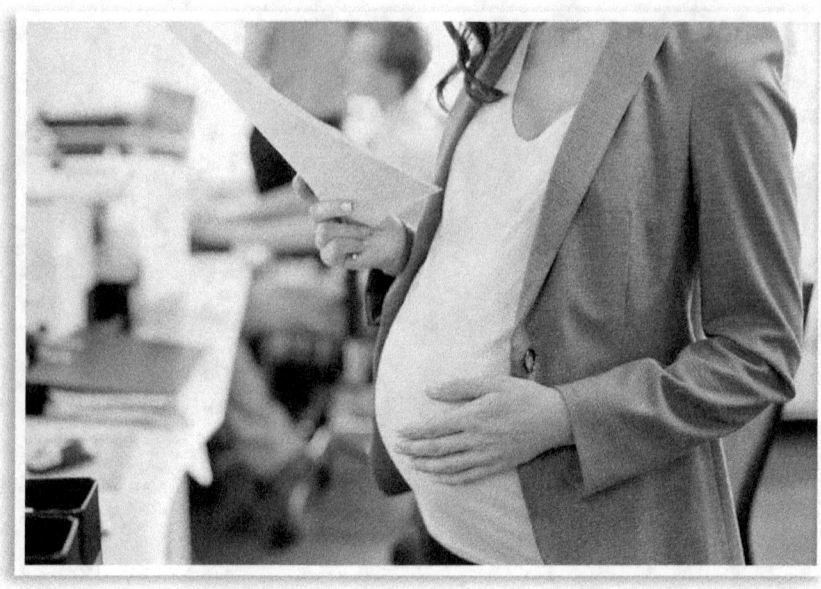

Even if you are planning on leaving your workplace, early on in the pregnancy is not the best time to mention this. Be sure to keep all of your options open and have all of your ducks in a row before you give your employer permission to cut your hours or start finding your replacement. After all, it's your right to continue working if you so choose.

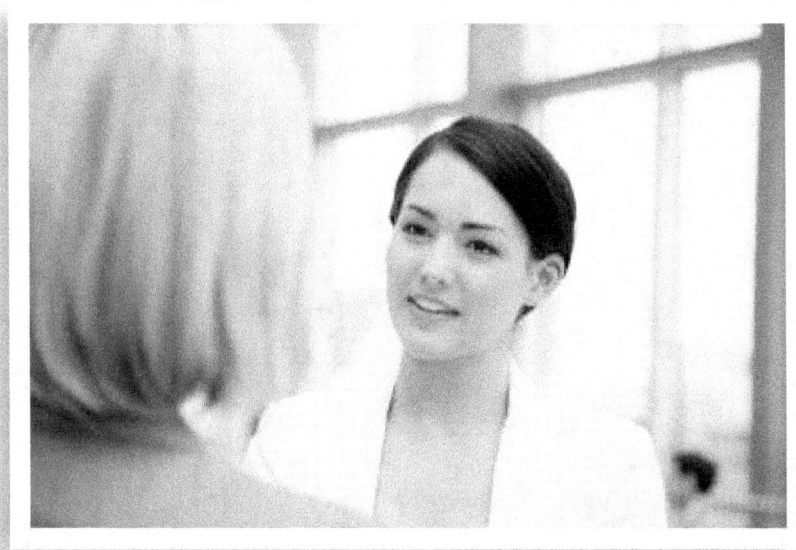

Pay attention to the rules of your company and the rights you have. Often, maternity pay is calculated based upon hours worked during the earliest part of your pregnancy, so make sure that you are making the best decisions for you and your family. Know who to talk to if your hours or wages get cut ahead of time.

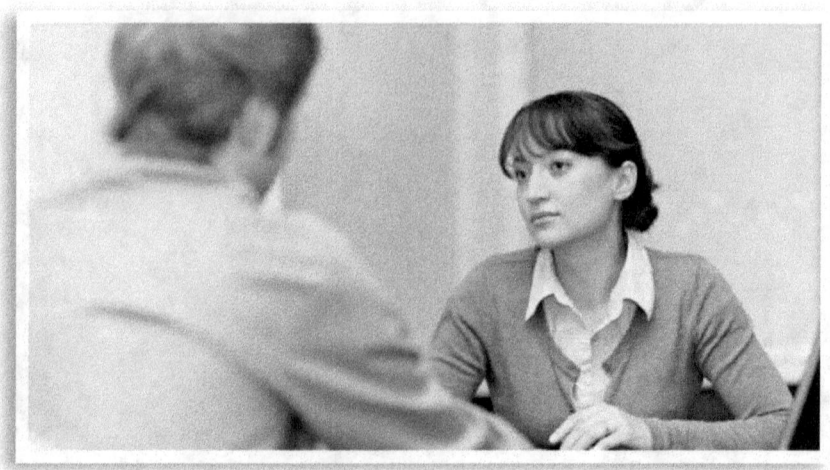

Don't be too nervous though. When you make the announcement you'll most likely be congratulated on the good news. After all, new babies are always great news! Plus, your employer should know that handling your pregnancy with grace will foster loyalty in you as an employee. Bottom line: be prepared, but don't sweat it!

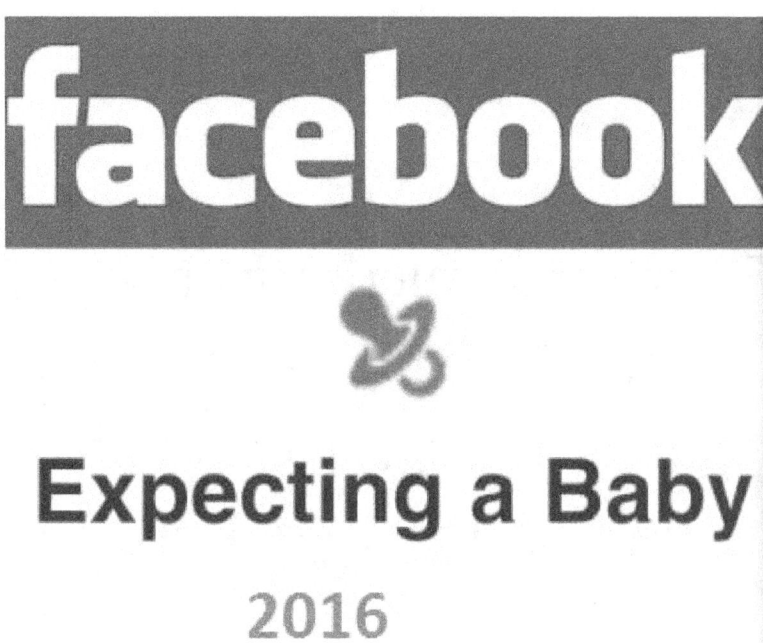

Expecting a Baby

2016

Now that your close friends and your coworkers are in on the joyous secret, it's time for the big reveal: Social Media! Remember to keep this one for last, as you don't want your family or your boss to think you're not being forthright with them.

There are a plethora of ways to reveal the big news to the public at large, so have some fun with this one. Here are some ideas for new mothers to make this exciting time extra fun:

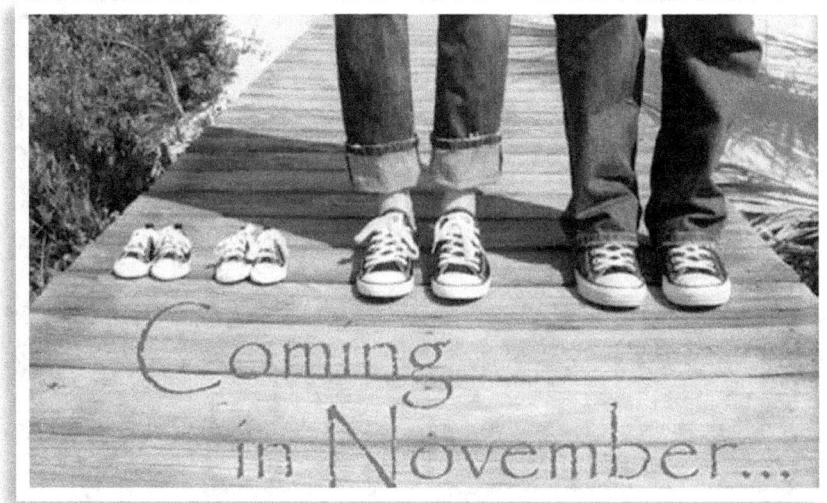

Coming in November...

Use the shoes: buy a pair of cute little baby shoes, and take a photo of them in between you and your partner's shoes. This is a classic way to intimate that you will soon have a few extra tiny feet around your house!

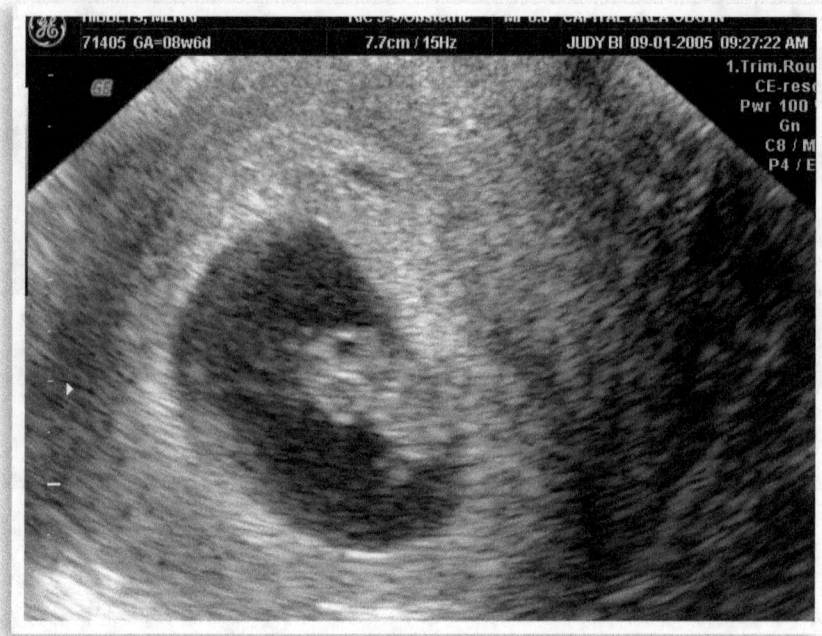

Share a baby scan: your first pictures of baby are very special, and a great way to get your point across immediately. After all, everyone recognizes an ultrasound picture, though they may not be able to distinguish of the proper parts and pieces. This one works best if you are able to capture the baby engaged in a cute in-womb baby habit, like sucking his thumb or sticking out his tongue!

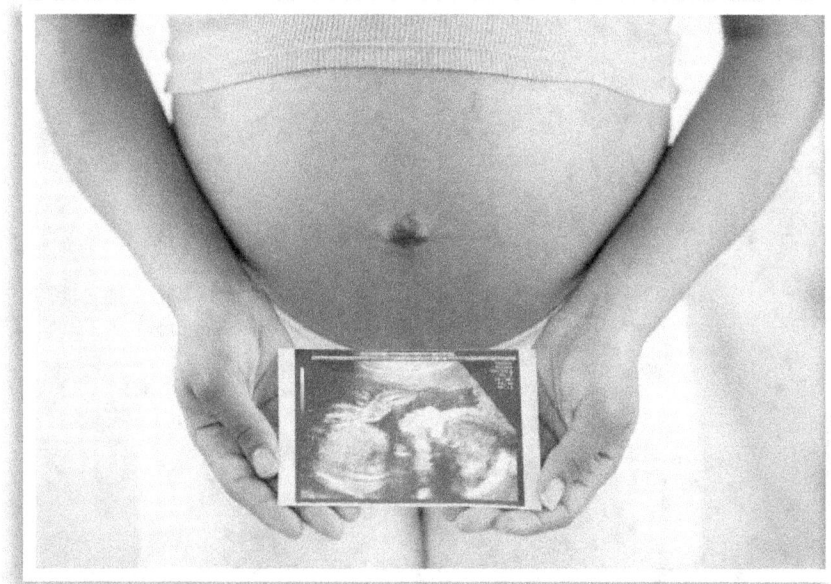

Film your test: though you may not reveal the film to the general public until a bit later, you can share the the joy of those first moments thanks to your handy smartphone. Watch as the results show on the test, and pan over to film your reactions. Record those first precious smiles and hugs to remember for yourselves, and to share with your friends and family.

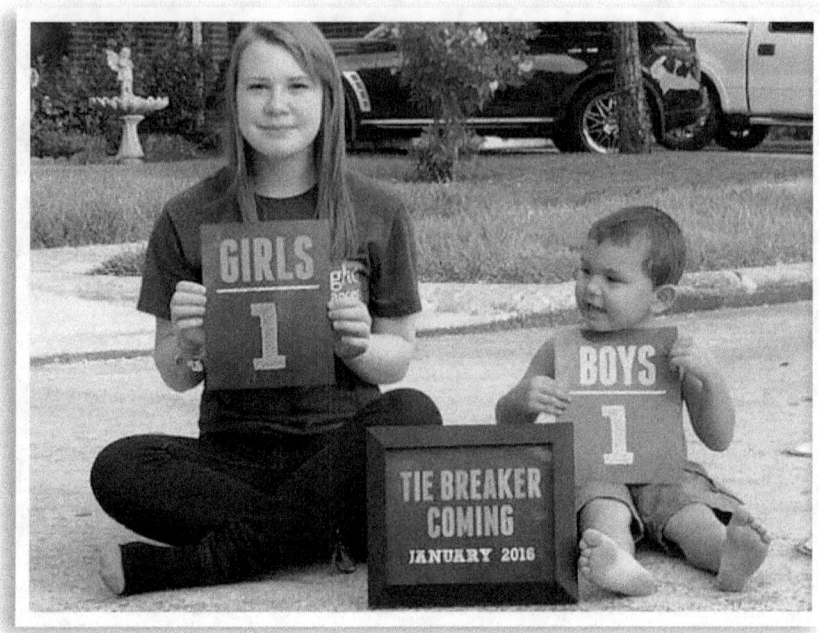

Sibling spill: have the soon to be big brother or sister tell the world! You can record a video of the big reveal, with them announcing your new addition. Or, grab them a super cute shirt they can wear with pride with the news and have themselves a brand-new celebrate baby present. It's a win-win for them, and they get to be the star.

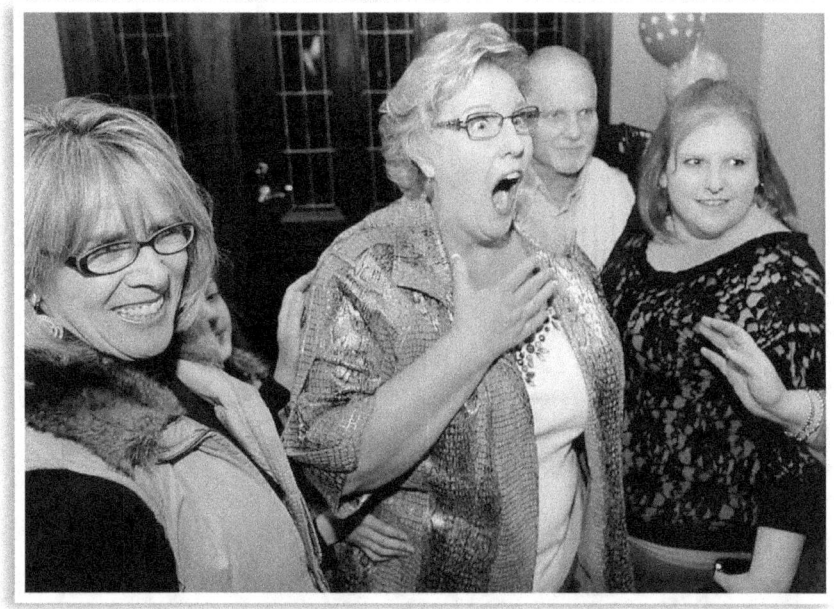

Film the family reaction: when you tell your parents that they are going to be grandparents, it's a big moment for everyone involved. Preserve the moment with a well-placed camera, and share it with the world. Who knows? There could be a very cute and funny moment to keep the masses entertained.

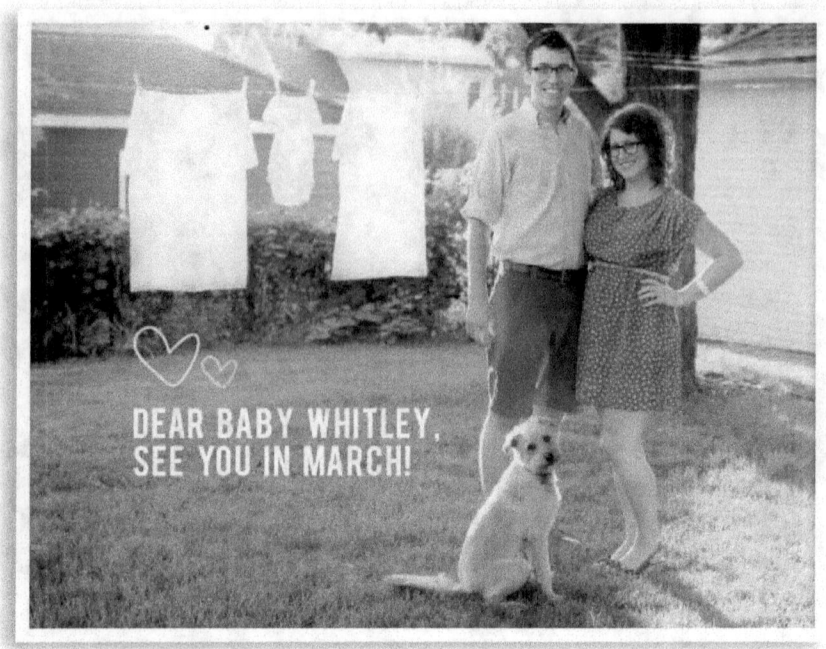

DEAR BABY WHITLEY,
SEE YOU IN MARCH!

A cute clothesline: all you need for a picture perfect pregnancy announcement is a cute baby onesie and a couple of adult sized t-shirts. Hang them in a row on a clothesline and you've got a classic and classy announcement. It's even a funny precursor to all of the laundry in your very near future (ok, maybe not so funny).

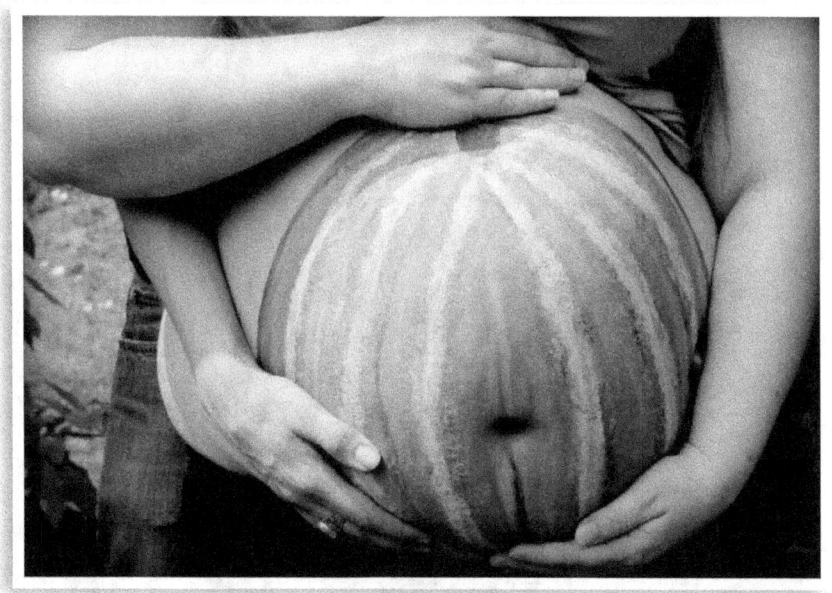

Painted belly: you can use a little body paint and reveal your soon-to-be much more swollen belly with the announcement. Tech savvy parents? Tell people how far along you are with a loading bar for how much longer you have to wait for baby's appearance.

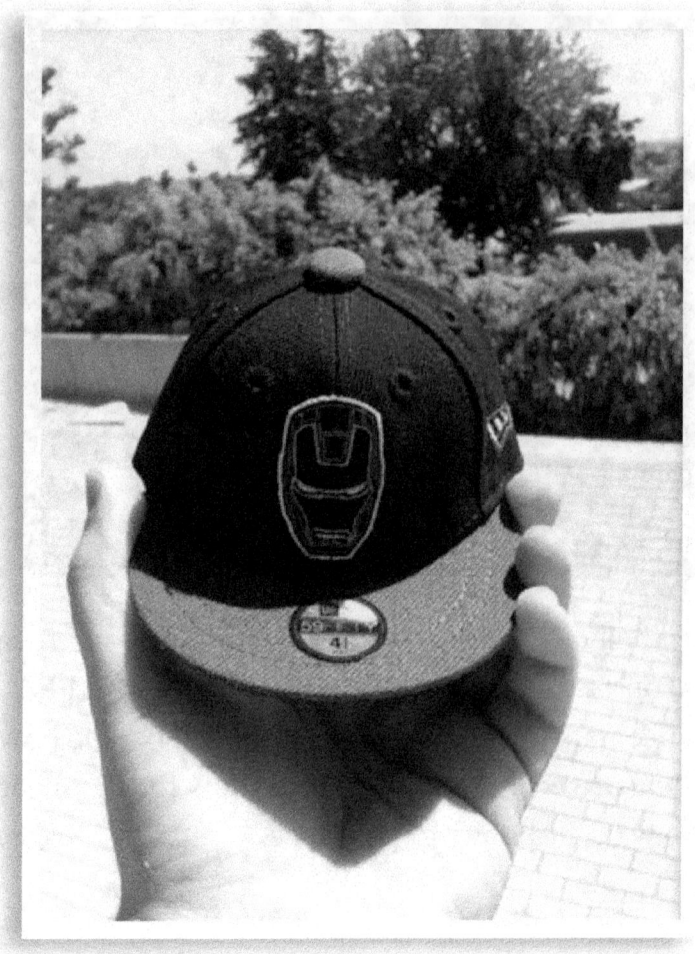

A holiday coming up? Celebrate the newest little gift in your life with a sweet gift hinting at the baby to be. Grab a baby sized ball cap with the fan's favorite sports team, or present daddy with a sippy cup, baby rattle, or other obvious baby item to announce the new big deal. A photo of father to be with baby items in hand and a big smile on his face is a great way to present your news to the world.

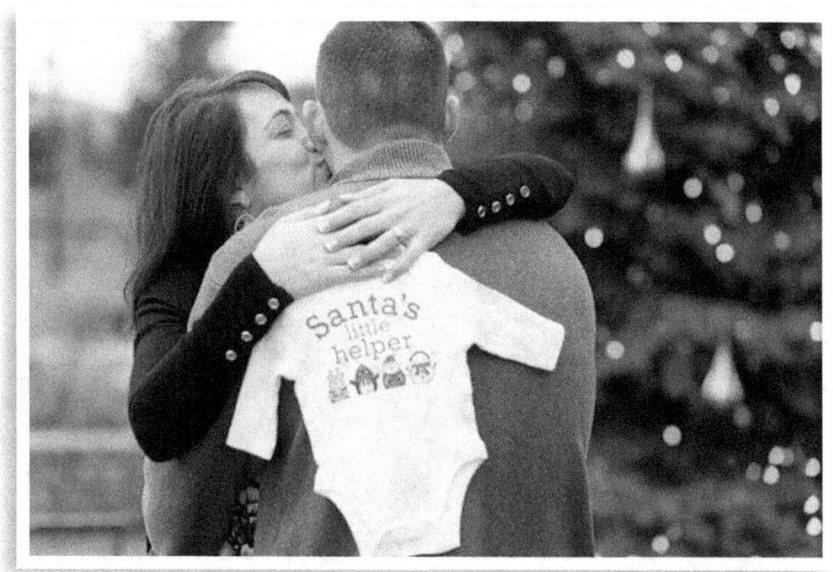

Show off your research skills. You're reading a bunch of pregnancy related material anyway, so snap a photo of you and your partner boning up on the new situation! The title on your tome will set the stage for all kinds of admiring comments for those who are paying close attention to your pics.

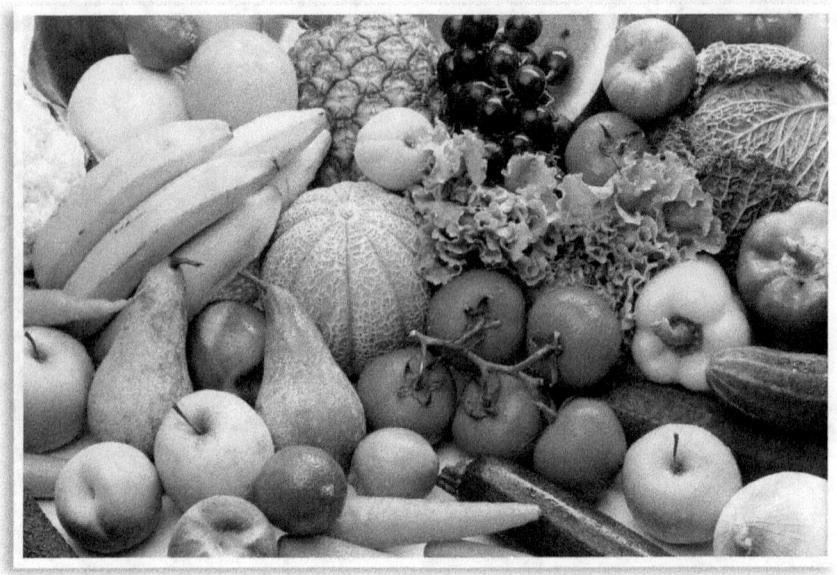

Share the size. Baby websites and apps provide us with all sorts of information about the progress of our infant's growth, so you can take a picture of the fruit or vegetable of the month and title it with a few fun facts about your fetus.

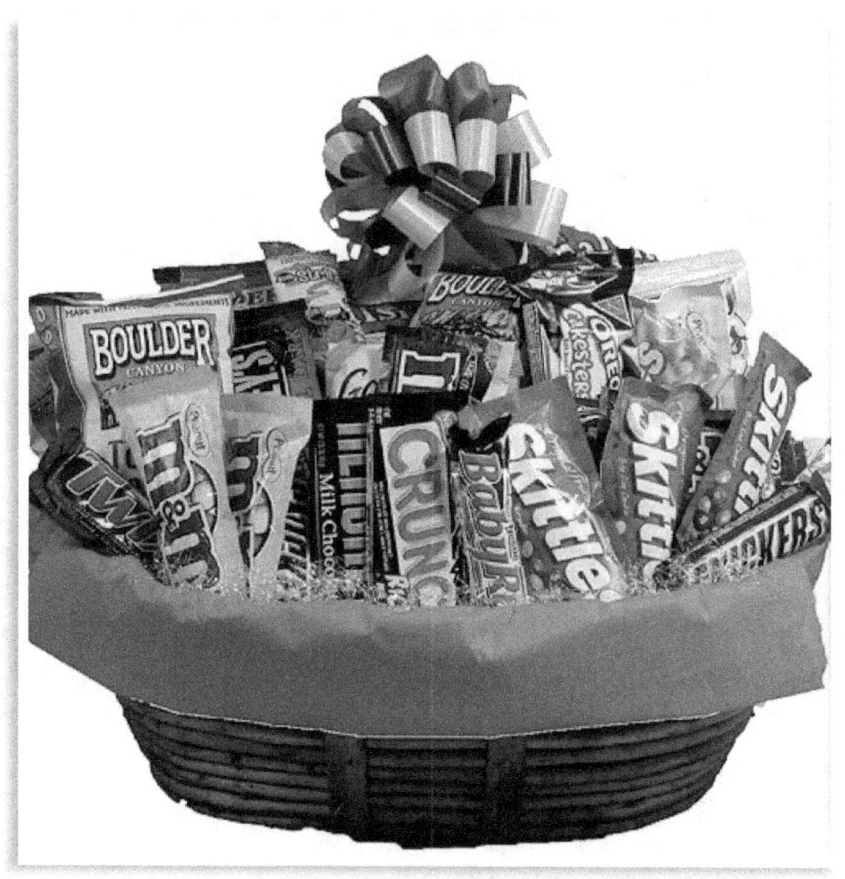

Customized sweets can be just the treat you need to get your point across. Order a lot of candies or chocolates that say something adorable like "Baby's Coming!" and pass small bags to friends and family when you see them. Not only will they convey your message, they'll bring a little bit of extra happiness to your news.

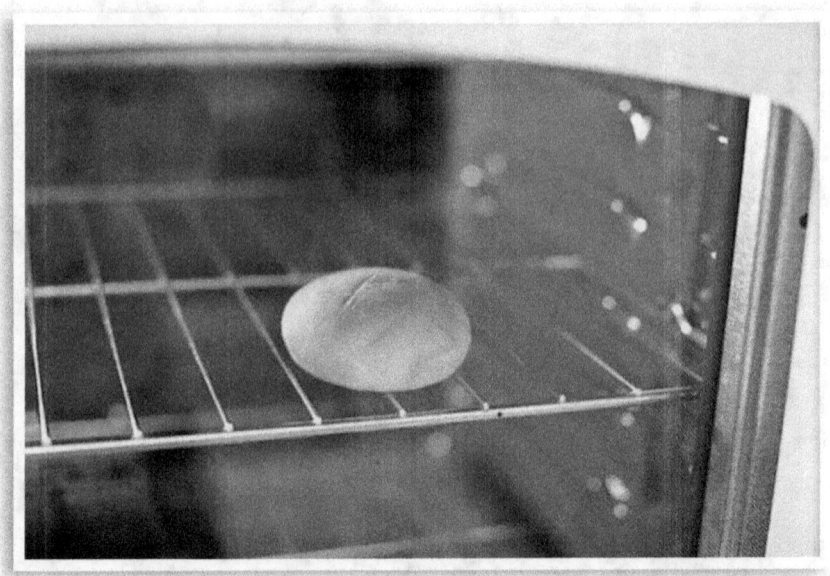

"A bun in the oven" can be more than just a turn of phrase: you can get to baking and take a quick snap of your snack! Serve the bun up to your honey, and then share the pic with your friends.

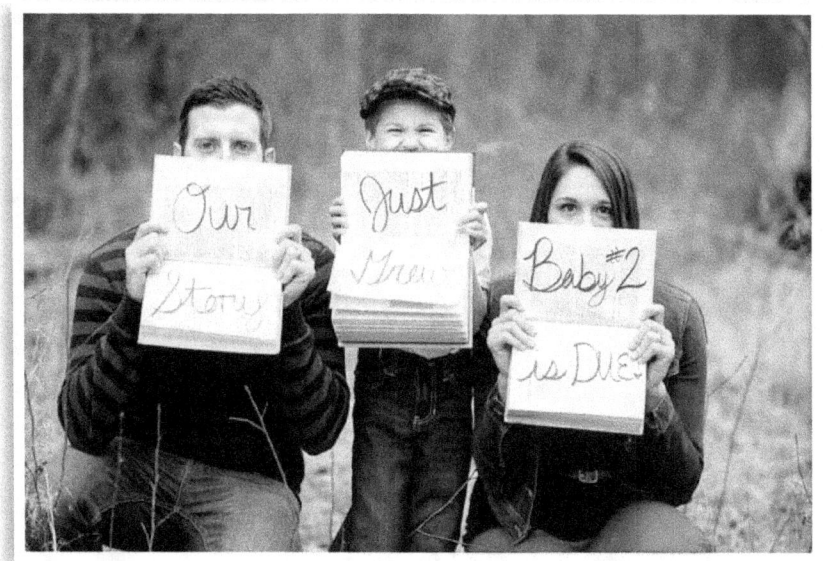

Family photo session: for some extra special protraits that you will treasure for a lifetime, consider booking a photo shoot with a professional photographer. You can reveal the baby news in a beautiful photo series, telling your story through perfect moments with proper lighting and fund backgrounds!

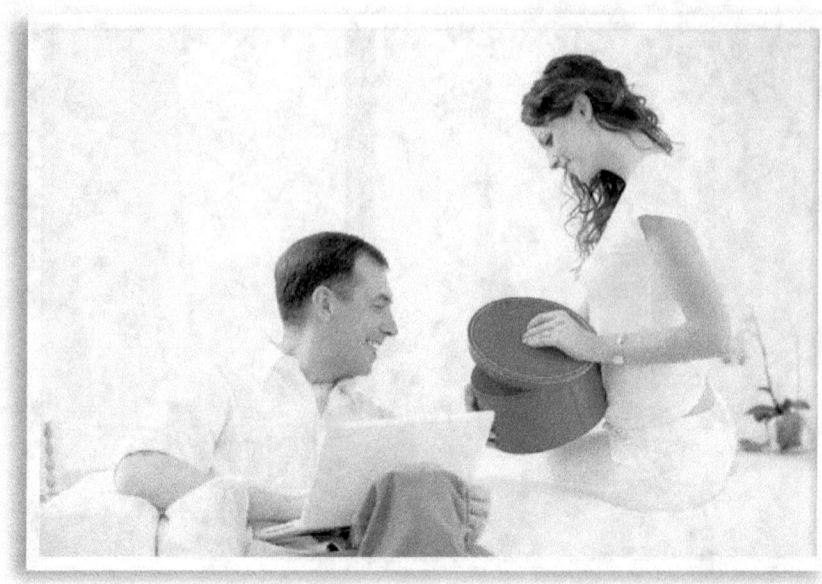

Father's day: the next time father's day rolls around and you're trying to get preggers, pick up a card for your man. Keep it hidden until the big day, then take photos of him opening up your "just because" surprise!

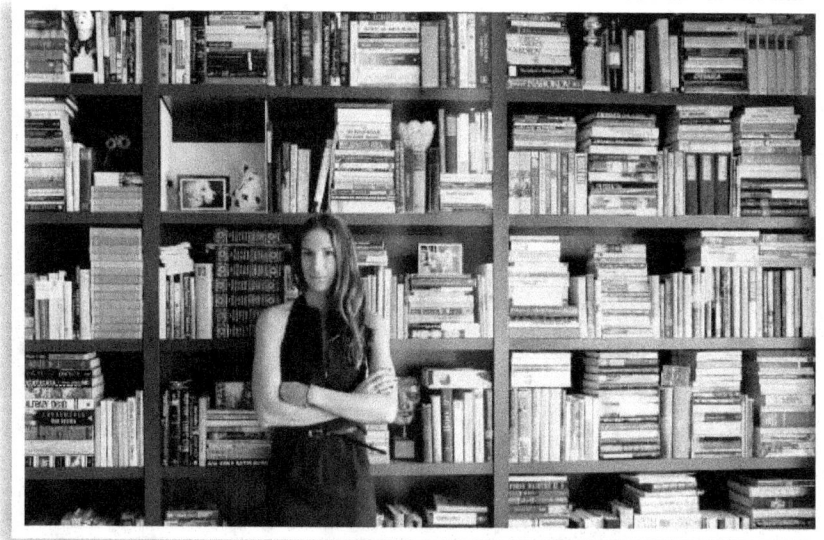

A little library: grab your favorite children's books to start baby's collection. You can take a photo of the shelf to share with your family and friends, indicating that your reading list will change once the due date rolls around.

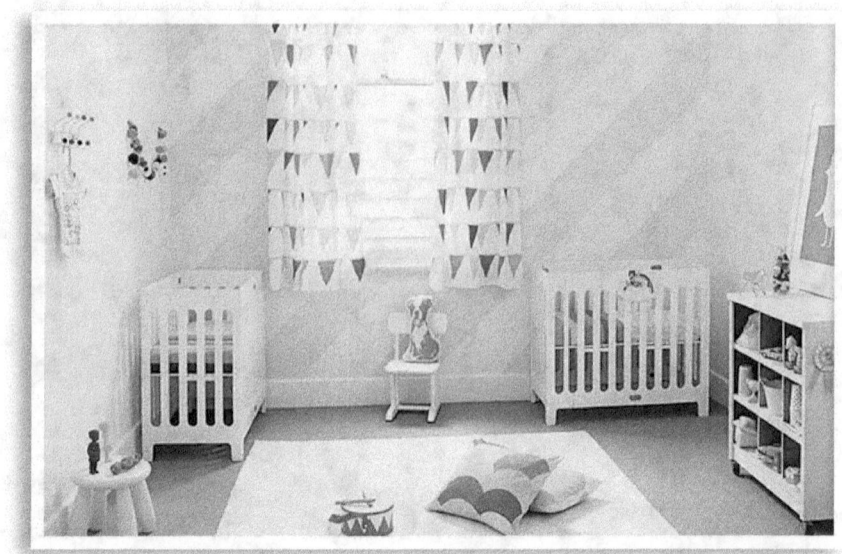

Nursery photos: Type 'A' mothers generally start outfitting the nursery right away. If this is you, take a photo of the crib or bassinette to let everyone know your bundle is on it's way! You can also set up a little vignette for your family with a teddy bear and some baby toys. Be sure to include your due date somewhere in the photo!

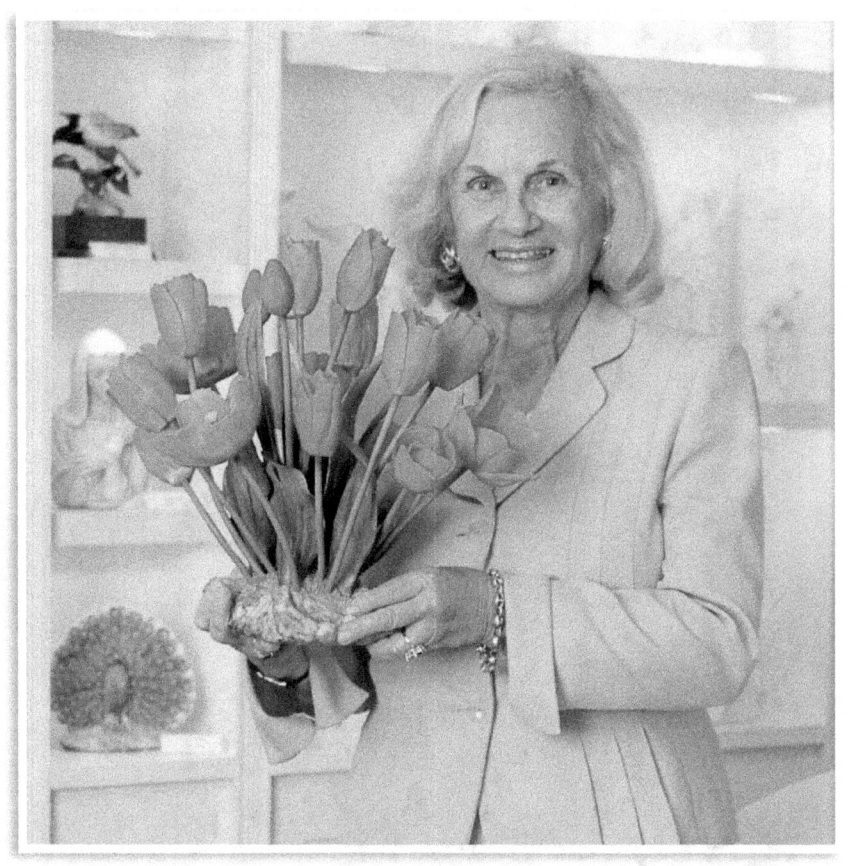

Flower power: you can present flowers at a family gathering with your special news tied around the stem. Make everyone feel special, and share the good news at the same time. Some mothers even opt to tie a rattle or a pacifier to the stem for an extra-cute treat.

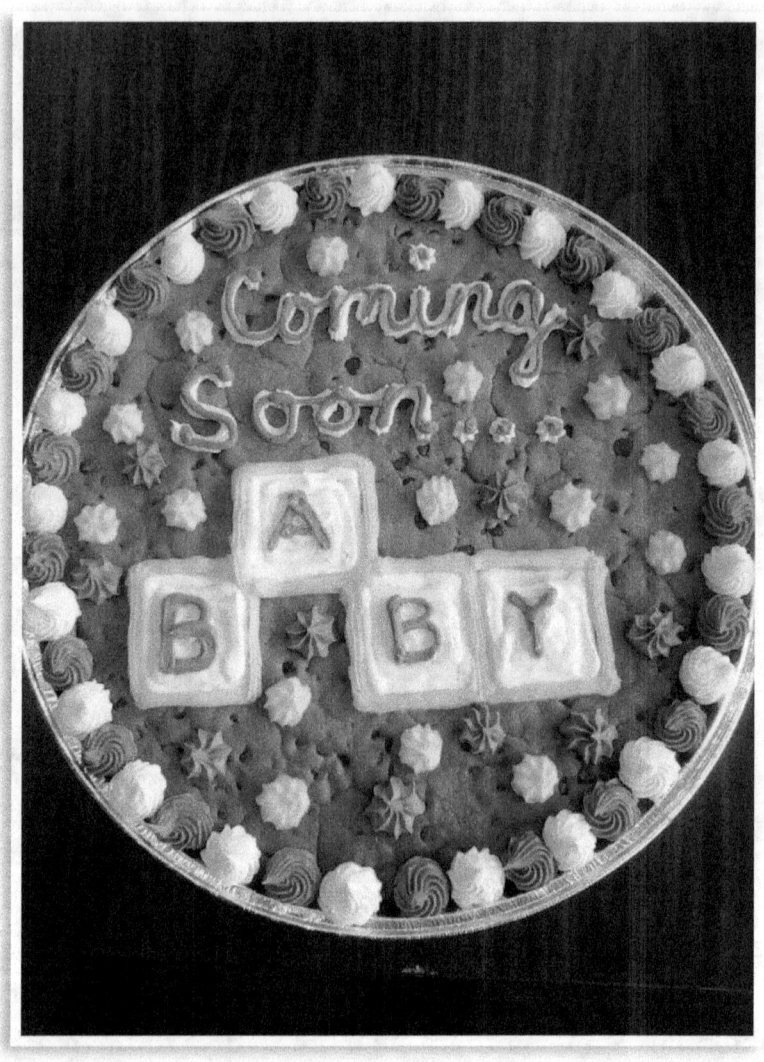

Nothing says good news like a cake! Take a snapshot when you surprise your family with the good news in the form of delicious decorative icing on your favorite flavor. Besides, you're probably craving a little bit of sweetness right about now anyway.

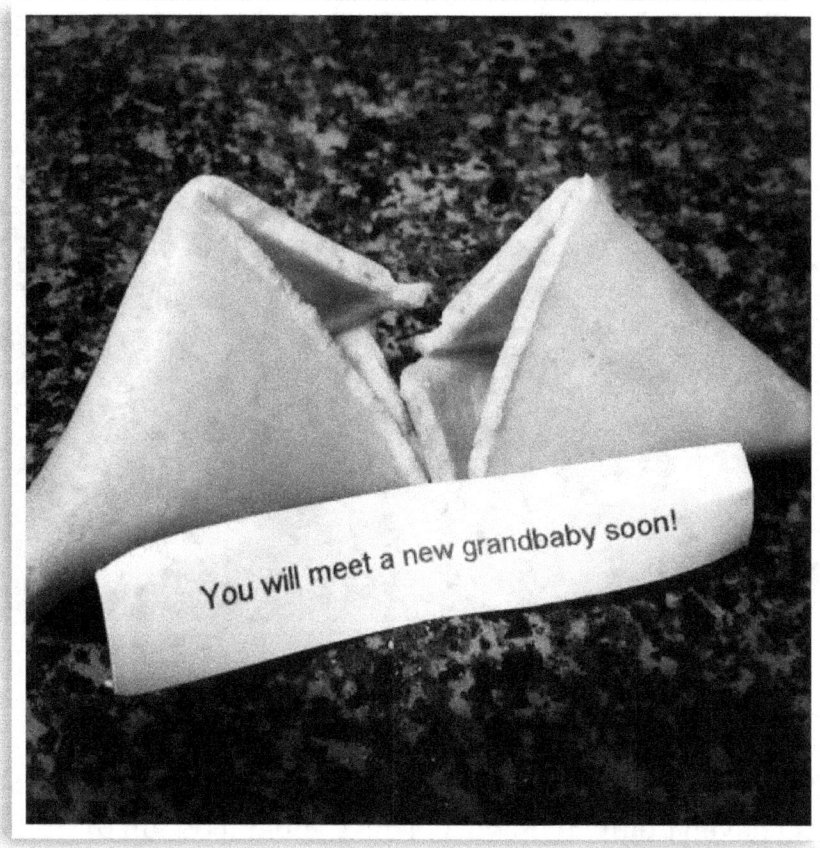

Fortune cookie fun: if you can wait for a custom order to arrive, head online and write a sweet message with the baby news to be inserted into a fortune cookie. You can tell your hubby or the grandma to be that you want to take them out for lunch, and that you'll bring a special dessert. It will be the sweetest treat they'll ever have.

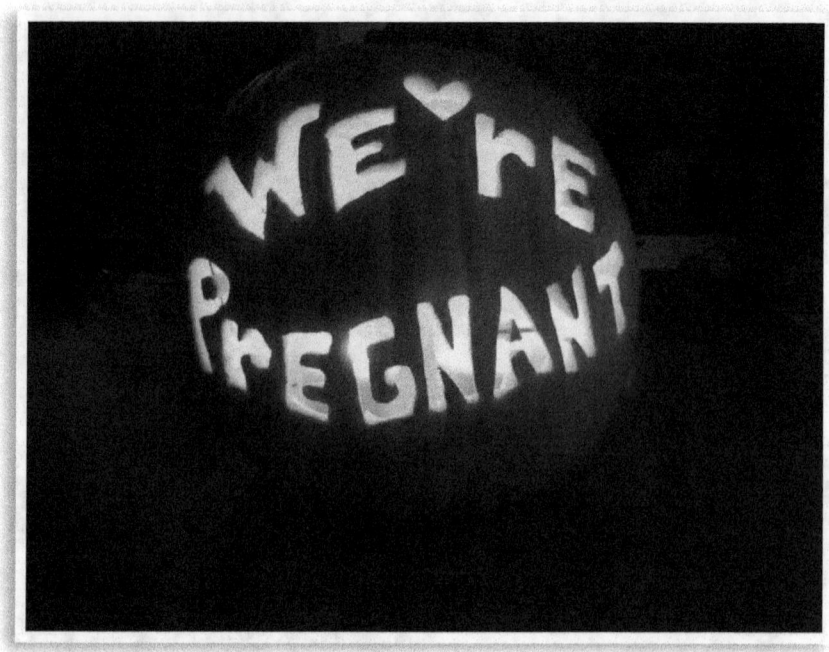

Use the 'we': a more subtle way to tell people you're pregnant is to begin using the royal "We" whenever you refer to yourself. The closest people to you will know that you haven't pinned down a prince, and it'll be fun to respond when they ask you what in the world you are talking about.

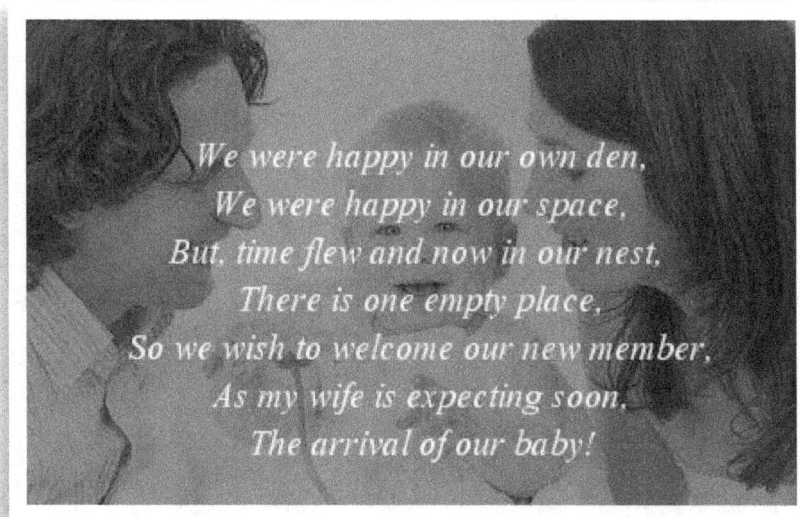

We were happy in our own den,
We were happy in our space,
But, time flew and now in our nest,
There is one empty place,
So we wish to welcome our new member,
As my wife is expecting soon,
The arrival of our baby!

Literary talent: Poetry is a sweet and sassy way to send your message, so try your hand at a little rhyme and span action. You can send this out in cards to your family, keep one for the albums, and share one on the internet. It's a fun triple use way to share your talent and the great news at the same time!

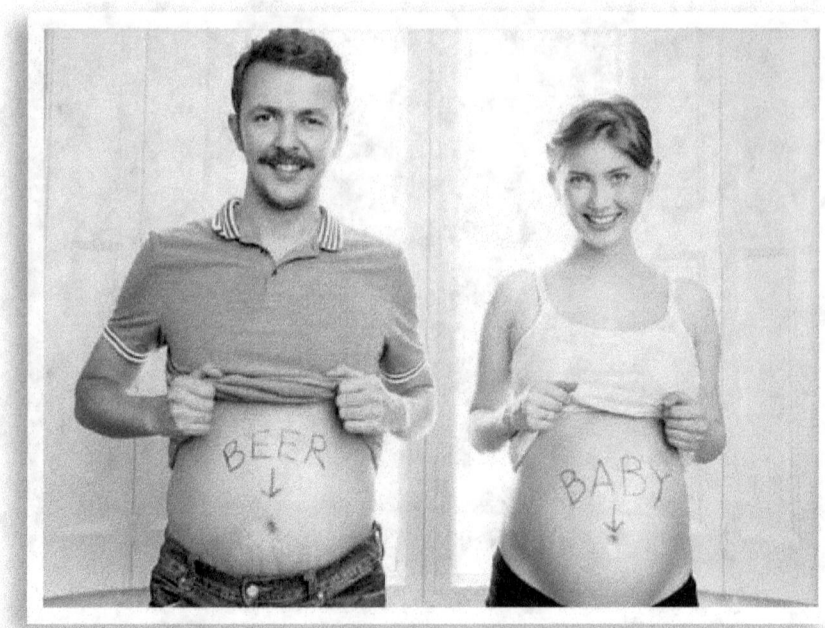

There are hundreds of ways to share your news, so put your own flair on it and have fun! This is an exciting time in your life. If you're new to motherhood, you are beginning a journey that will forever change you and your life in innumerable ways. If this is a new addition to an already happy family with youngsters, everyone is will be thrilled to get to know the new sibling. Make the beginning of this journey as fun as possible. There is a lot more joy to come!

Thank You!

We hope you enjoyed the book! All pictures and words were lovingly put together by experts who really love what they do! We really hope you learned something new today!

We would really appreciate it, if you could PLEASE take the time to let us know how we're doing by leaving a review on the Amazon website. We appreciate any comments you may have – what you enjoyed about the book, what additions you would have liked to have seen and what you would like to see in future publications.

Any comments will help understand better what you and your kids most enjoy and allows us to better provide exactly what you want!

Thought Junction Publishing

A NOTE FROM THE WRITER

Sam's life revolves around her family, devoted mother of 3 - Noah (6), Oscar (3) and Poppy (11months) - she writes in a real way, aiming to answer the questions that other books don't cover, to fill in the blanks and inform parents and parents-to-be of the truth about raising children in the modern world.

Sam's writings emphasize that the readers are not alone - that there is a community of support available, and other people to talk to who can help, support and assist.

When she's not writing books, Sam is an advisor and avid blogger for Ideal Parent - http://ideal-parent.com - spreading support, care and advice across the web!

Join Sam on Ideal Parent and keep an eye out for her books - she's on a mission to help parents worldwide - join her and spread the word!